Erotic Positions and Techniques

"A Step-by-Step Kama Sutra Guide for Couples"

PETER MILLER

Introduction
Chapter 1
    Introduction to the Kama Sutra
Chapter 2
    Preparing for Intimacy
Chapter 3
    Basic Positions and Techniques
Chapter 4
    Intermediate Positions and Techniques
Chapter 5
    Advanced Positions and Techniques
Chapter 6
    Emotional and Spiritual Aspects of Intimacy
Chapter 7
    Troubleshooting Common Challenges
Chapter 8
    Conclusion and Next Steps

Introduction

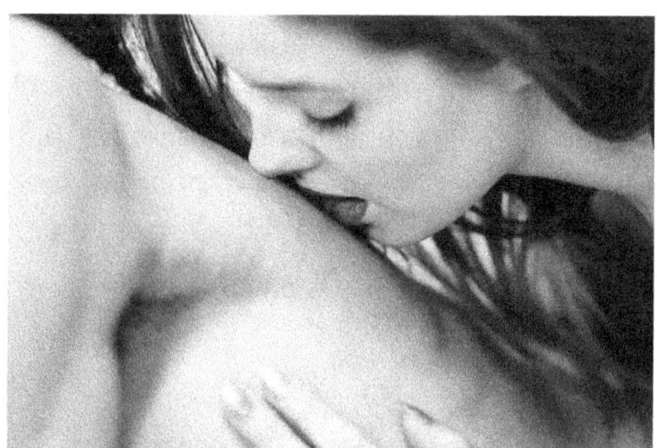

Intimacy is a vital part of a healthy relationship, and exploring new ways to connect with your partner can bring you closer together. The ancient Indian text, Kama Sutra, is known for its rich insights into the art of lovemaking and has been a source of inspiration for couples around the world for centuries.

In this book, "Erotic Positions and Techniques: A Step-by-Step Kama Sutra Guide for Couples," we delve into the depths of the Kama Sutra to provide a comprehensive guide for couples seeking to deepen their intimacy and explore new levels of pleasure.

With detailed descriptions and illustrations, we take you through a step-by-step journey of the most sensual and erotic positions and techniques from the Kama Sutra. From classic positions like the "Lotus" and the "Cowgirl" to more advanced techniques like the "Splitting of a Bamboo" and the "Crab Walk," you will discover new ways to connect with your partner and experience mind-blowing pleasure.

But this book is not just about physical techniques; it also explores the emotional and spiritual aspects of lovemaking. We provide guidance on how to create a sacred and intimate space, how to communicate your desires and needs, and how to cultivate a deeper connection with your partner.

Whether you are a beginner or an experienced couple seeking to deepen your intimacy, this book will guide you on a journey of discovery and exploration. So, let us embark on this journey together, and discover the rich and sensual world of the Kama Sutra.

Chapter 1

Introduction to the Kama Sutra

The Kama Sutra is an ancient Indian text that has been celebrated for its insights into the art of lovemaking for centuries. Its origin dates back to the 2nd century CE, and it was written by the sage Vatsyayana. The Kama Sutra is divided into seven books, which cover a wide range of topics related to human sexuality, including positions, techniques, and attitudes towards sex. While the Kama Sutra is often associated with physical positions and techniques, it also emphasizes the importance of emotional and spiritual aspects of lovemaking.

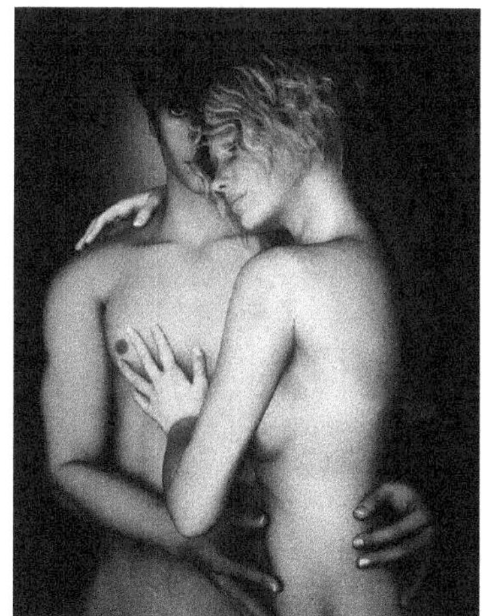

The significance of the Kama Sutra lies in its comprehensive exploration of human sexuality. The text recognizes that sex is a natural part of life and acknowledges that there is much to be learned about the nuances of lovemaking. The Kama Sutra is not just a guide to physical positions and techniques; it also provides a framework for understanding the emotional and spiritual aspects of intimacy.

At its core, the Kama Sutra is about connection and pleasure. It recognizes that sex is not just about reproduction but is also an expression of love, intimacy, and pleasure. Through its teachings, the Kama Sutra encourages couples to explore their desires and connect with each other on a deeper level.

Understanding the principles of the Kama Sutra is essential for couples seeking to deepen their intimacy. The Kama Sutra is not just a manual of positions and techniques but a comprehensive guide to the art of lovemaking. It emphasizes the importance of communication, respect, and mutual pleasure. By following the principles of the Kama Sutra, couples can create a safe and intimate space where they can explore their desires and connect with each other on a deeper level.

The role of intimacy in a relationship cannot be overstated. Intimacy is the glue that binds couples together, and it is the foundation of a healthy relationship. Intimacy encompasses both physical and

6

emotional connection and involves trust, vulnerability, and mutual respect. The Kama Sutra recognizes the importance of intimacy in a relationship and provides a roadmap for couples seeking to deepen their connection.

In conclusion, the Kama Sutra is an ancient Indian text that has been celebrated for its insights into the art of lovemaking for centuries. It emphasizes the importance of physical, emotional, and spiritual aspects of intimacy and encourages couples to explore their desires and connect with each other on a deeper level. By understanding the principles of the Kama Sutra and the role of intimacy in a relationship, couples can create a safe and intimate space where they can explore their desires and deepen their connection.

Chapter 2

Preparing for Intimacy

Intimacy is an essential part of any healthy relationship, and creating a safe and intimate space is essential for a fulfilling sexual experience. Preparing for intimacy involves more than just physical preparation; it also involves emotional and mental preparation. In this chapter, we will explore how to create a sacred and intimate space, communicate with your partner, and prepare yourself emotionally and physically for intimacy.

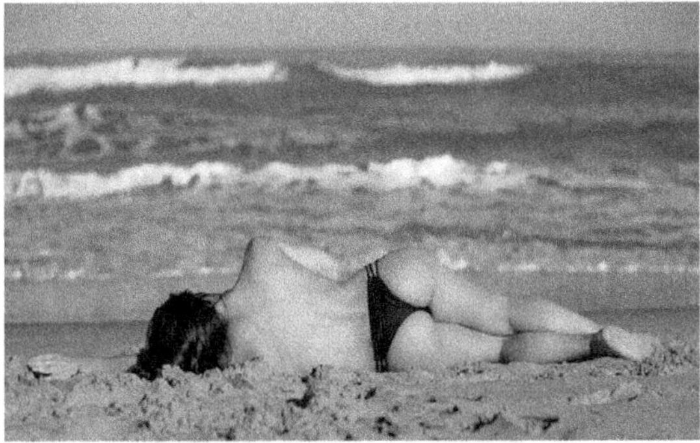

Creating a Sacred and Intimate Space

Creating a sacred and intimate space is essential for a fulfilling sexual experience. The environment in which you make love can impact your mood, emotions, and level of relaxation. Therefore, it is important to create a comfortable and safe environment for intimacy. Here are some tips for creating a sacred and intimate space:

- **Choose the right location:** When choosing a location for intimacy, consider a space where you and your partner feel comfortable and relaxed. This could be your bedroom, a hotel room, or even a private spot in nature. Ensure that the space is clean, comfortable, and free from distractions.

- **Set the mood:** Create a romantic ambiance by using soft lighting, candles, or music. Scented candles or incense can also help create a relaxing and sensual atmosphere.

- **Clear your mind:** Before engaging in intimacy, it is important to clear your mind and let go of any stress or distractions. You can practice deep breathing, meditation, or visualization to relax your mind and body.

- **Use props:** Introducing props like pillows, blankets, or even sex toys can enhance your sexual experience and create a more comfortable and enjoyable space.

Communicating with Your Partner

Communication is essential for any healthy relationship, and it is especially important when it comes to intimacy. Good communication can help you and your partner feel more comfortable, relaxed, and connected during intimacy. Here are some tips for communicating with your partner:

- **Share your desires:** Let your partner know what you like and what turns you on. This can help you both explore your desires and enhance your sexual experience.

- **Be open and honest:** If you are feeling anxious, nervous, or uncomfortable, it is important to communicate this to your partner. This can help you both work together to create a safe and comfortable environment for intimacy.

- Listen to your partner: It is important to listen to your partner and be attentive to their needs and desires. This can help you both connect on a deeper level and enhance your sexual experience.

- **Use nonverbal communication:** Nonverbal communication, such as touch, eye contact, or body language, can also help you and your partner connect on a deeper level during intimacy.

Preparing Yourself Emotionally and Physically

Preparing yourself emotionally and physically for intimacy is essential for a fulfilling sexual experience. Here are some tips for preparing yourself emotionally and physically:

- **Manage stress:** Stress can interfere with intimacy and affect your overall well-being. Practice stress-management techniques like meditation, deep breathing, or exercise to help you relax and feel more at ease.

- **Practice self-care:** Taking care of yourself physically and mentally can help you feel more confident and comfortable during intimacy. Get enough sleep, eat a healthy diet, and engage in activities that make you feel happy and relaxed.

- **Explore your body:** Understanding your own body and what feels good for you can help you communicate your desires to your partner and enhance your sexual experience.

- **Consider therapy:** If you have any underlying emotional or psychological issues that are affecting your ability to be intimate, consider seeking the help of a therapist or counselor.

Conclusion

Preparing for intimacy involves more than just physical preparation; it also involves emotional and mental preparation. Creating a sacred and intimate space, communicating with your partner, and preparing yourself emotionally and physically are all essential components of preparing for intimacy.

Chapter 3

Basic Positions and Techniques

Sexual positions and techniques play a crucial role in enhancing your sexual experience. The Kama Sutra offers a variety of positions and techniques to help you and your partner connect on a deeper level and experience greater pleasure. In this chapter, we will explore some of the basic positions and techniques that are commonly used in the Kama Sutra.

The "Lotus" Position

The Lotus position is a classic Kama Sutra position that involves sitting facing each other with your legs crossed and your arms around each other. This position allows for deep eye contact and intimate touching, making it a great choice for couples who want to connect on a deeper emotional level.

To get into the Lotus position, sit cross-legged facing your partner. Place your hands on your partner's shoulders, and have your partner do the same. Lean forward and kiss each other, and then slowly rock back and forth in sync with each other's movements.

The "Yawning" Position

The Yawning position is a relaxed and comfortable position that involves lying side by side with your legs intertwined. This position is great for couples who want to cuddle and feel close to each other.

To get into the Yawning position, lie down on your side facing your partner. Place your top leg over your partner's leg, and your bottom leg between your partner's legs. Your arms can either be wrapped around your partner or resting at your sides.

The "Missionary" Position

The Missionary position is one of the most popular sexual positions and involves the man on top of the woman. This position allows for deep penetration and intimate touching, making it a great choice for couples who want to connect on a physical and emotional level.

To get into the Missionary position, the woman lies on her back with her legs spread apart. The man then kneels or lies on top of her and enters her from above. The woman can wrap her legs around the man's waist or keep them straight.

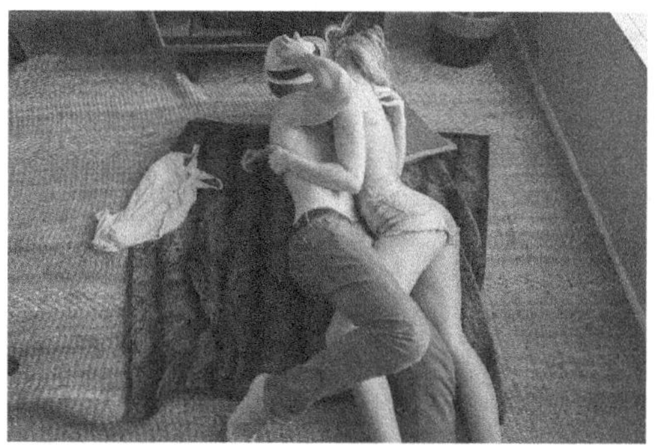

The "Doggy Style" Position

The Doggy Style position is a popular position that involves the woman on all fours with the man behind her. This position allows for deep penetration and can be very stimulating for both partners.

To get into the Doggy Style position, the woman gets down on her hands and knees with her legs apart. The man then enters her from behind and can either kneel or stand behind her. The woman can arch her back or rest on her elbows to adjust the angle of penetration.

The "Cowgirl" Position

The Cowgirl position involves the woman on top of the man, facing him. This position allows the woman to take control and set the pace, making it a great choice for couples who want to switch things up and explore new sensations.

To get into the Cowgirl position, the man lies on his back with his legs apart. The woman straddles him, facing him, and lowers herself onto him. The woman can either place her hands on the man's chest or rest them on his legs for support.

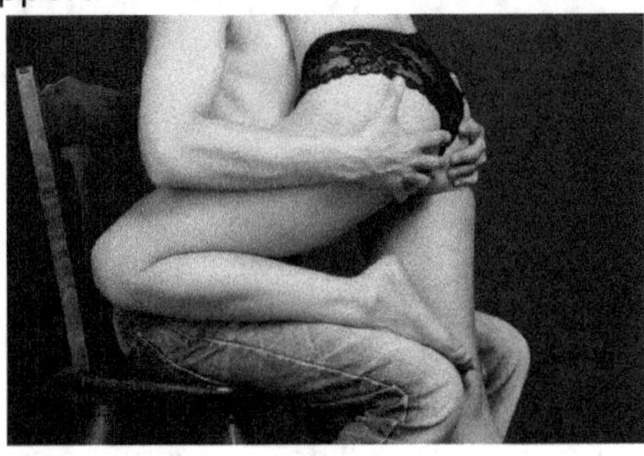

The "Reverse Cowgirl" Position

The Reverse Cowgirl position is similar to the Cowgirl position, but with the woman facing away from the man. This position allows for deep penetration and can be very stimulating for both partners.

To get into the Reverse Cowgirl position, the man lies on his back with his legs apart. The woman straddles him, facing away from him, and lowers herself onto him. The woman can place her hands on the man's legs or rest them on his chest for support.

In addition to trying different positions and techniques, communication is key to a fulfilling sexual experience. Don't be afraid to talk to your partner about what you like and what you don't like. Communication can help you and your partner understand each other's needs and desires and lead to a more satisfying sexual experience.

It's also important to remember that sexual pleasure is not just about the physical act of sex. Emotional and mental connection also plays a crucial role in enhancing sexual pleasure. Taking the time to connect with your partner on an emotional level outside of the bedroom can lead to a more fulfilling sexual experience inside the bedroom.

Lastly, it's important to prioritize safety during sexual activity. Using protection and getting tested regularly can help prevent the spread of sexually transmitted infections and unwanted pregnancies.

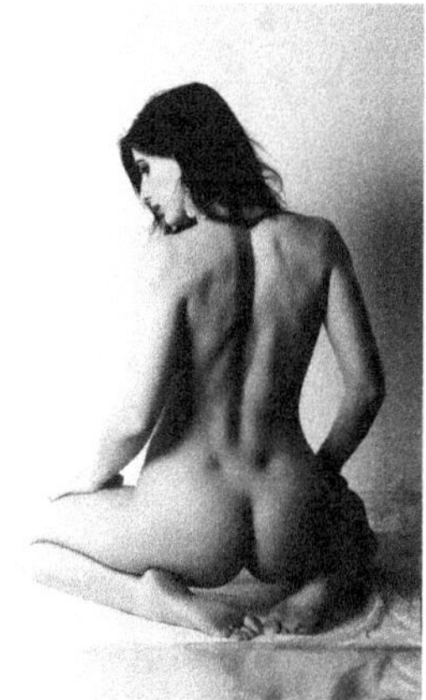

Conclusion

Exploring different sexual positions and techniques can help you and your partner connect on a deeper emotional and physical level. The Lotus, Yawning,

Missionary, Doggy Style, Cowgirl, and Reverse Cowgirl positions are just a few options available in the Kama Sutra. Remember to communicate with your partner, prioritize emotional and mental connection, and prioritize safety during sexual activity.

Chapter 4

Intermediate Positions and Techniques

In the Kama Sutra, there are a variety of sexual positions and techniques for couples to explore. As couples become more comfortable with the basic positions and techniques, they may want to explore intermediate positions and techniques to enhance their sexual experience. In this chapter, we will explore six intermediate positions and techniques: the Crab Walk, Crouching Tiger, Splitting of a Bamboo, Suspended Congress, Indrani, and Widely Opened.

The Crab Walk Position

The Crab Walk position is an intermediate position that requires a fair amount of strength and flexibility. The position involves the man sitting on the floor with his legs extended and his hands behind him to support his weight. The woman sits in the man's lap facing him, with her legs wrapped around his waist and her hands on his shoulders. The woman then leans back and supports herself with her hands on the floor behind her. This position allows for deep penetration and intimacy between the couple.

To perform the Crab Walk position, it's important to have good upper body strength and flexibility. This position can be challenging for some couples, but with practice and patience, it can become a favorite position.

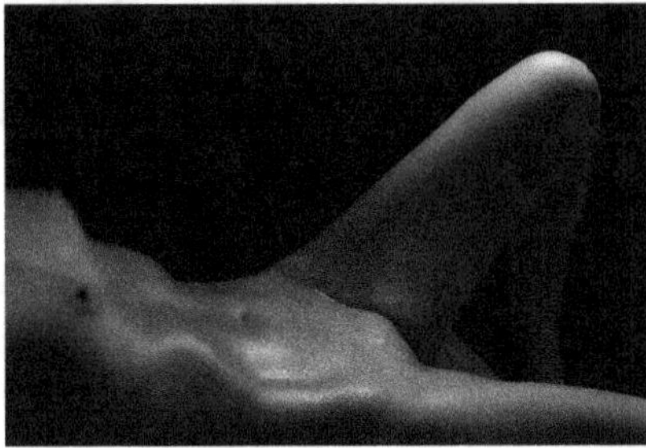

The Crouching Tiger Position

The Crouching Tiger position is another intermediate position that requires a bit of strength and flexibility. This position involves the woman lying on her back with her legs in the air, bent at the knees. The man then kneels between the woman's legs and holds onto her thighs, lifting her legs higher into the air. The woman can then wrap her legs around the man's waist, allowing for deep penetration and intimacy.

The Crouching Tiger position is great for couples who enjoy deep penetration and intimate contact. However, it can be a bit challenging for those who are not as flexible. It's important to take things slow and communicate with your partner during this position to avoid any discomfort.

The Splitting of a Bamboo Position

The Splitting of a Bamboo position is an intermediate position that requires a bit of balance and coordination. This position involves the man sitting on the floor with his legs extended and slightly apart. The woman then sits on top of the man facing away from him, with her legs wrapped around his waist. The woman then leans forward and places her hands on the floor between the man's legs, while the man holds onto her hips for support. This position allows for deep penetration and intimate contact between the couple.

The Splitting of a Bamboo position can be challenging for some couples due to the balance required. However, it can be a great way to switch things up and add some excitement to your sex life.

The Suspended Congress Position

The Suspended Congress position is an intermediate position that requires a bit of strength and coordination. This position involves the woman lying on her back with her legs in the air, while the man holds onto her ankles and lifts her legs into the air. The man then kneels between the woman's legs and enters her, allowing for deep penetration and intimate contact.

The Suspended Congress position is great for couples who enjoy deep penetration and intimate contact. However, it can be a bit challenging for those who are not as strong or coordinated. It's important to take things slow and communicate with your partner during this position to avoid any discomfort.

The Indrani Position

The Indrani position is an intermediate position that requires a bit of strength and flexibility. This position involves the woman lying on her back with her legs in the air and bent at the knees. The man then kneels between the woman's legs and holds onto her ankles, pulling her legs up and towards his chest. The woman can then wrap her legs around the man's waist, allowing for deep penetration and intimate contact.

The Indrani position can be challenging for some couples, but it can be incredibly rewarding for those who are willing to give it a try. It requires a certain level of strength and flexibility, but it can also be adjusted to accommodate different levels of physical ability. For example, the woman can use pillows or cushions to prop up her hips and make the position more comfortable.

One of the benefits of the Indrani position is that it allows for deep penetration, which can stimulate the G-spot and provide intense pleasure for the woman. It also allows for intimate eye contact between partners, which can deepen the emotional connection during sex.

To get into the Indrani position, the woman should lie on her back with her knees bent and her feet flat on the bed. The man can then kneel between her legs and lift her ankles, bringing her legs up towards his chest. He can then enter her while holding onto her ankles and allowing her to wrap her legs around his waist. The couple can adjust the angle of penetration by changing the height of the woman's hips with pillows or cushions.

As with any new position, it's important to communicate with your partner and take things slow at first. Make sure you're both comfortable and that you're not putting too much strain on any particular muscle groups. You may also want to experiment with different angles and levels of penetration to find what works best for both partners.

The Widely Opened position

The Widely Opened position is another intermediate position that can provide intense pleasure for both partners. In this position, the woman lies on her back with her legs spread wide apart. The man then kneels between her legs and enters her, holding onto her ankles or placing them over his shoulders for deeper penetration.

The Widely Opened position allows for deep penetration and stimulation of the G-spot, and it also provides the man with a great view of his partner's body. This can be incredibly erotic and can increase the emotional connection between partners.

To get into the Widely Opened position, the woman should lie on her back with her legs spread wide apart.

The man can then kneel between her legs and enter her, holding onto her ankles or placing them over his shoulders. The couple can experiment with different angles and levels of penetration to find what works best for them.

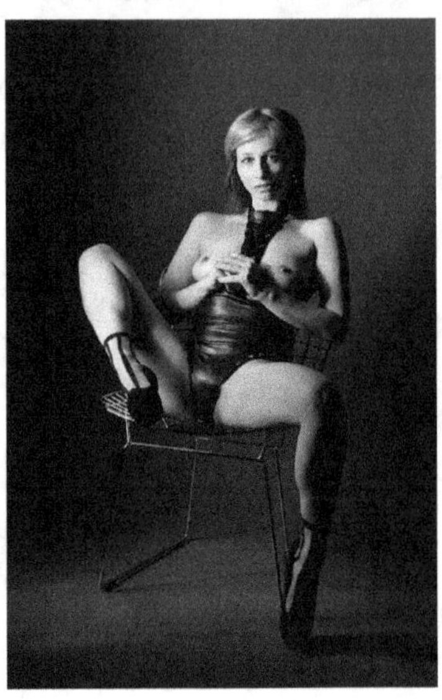

Chapter 5

Advanced Positions and Techniques

By this point, you and your partner have likely explored a range of sexual positions and techniques. If you're ready for a challenge and are looking to spice things up even more, advanced positions and techniques may be just what you need.

It's important to note that advanced positions and techniques may not be suitable for everyone. They may require a higher level of strength, flexibility, and coordination, and could potentially be uncomfortable or even painful if not executed properly. It's important to communicate with your partner, start slowly, and listen to your body to ensure that you are both comfortable and safe.

Here are six advanced positions and techniques to consider trying:

1. The "Mighty Wind" position

The Mighty Wind position is a variation of the traditional "Reverse Cowgirl" position that requires a significant amount of strength and flexibility. The woman straddles the man's hips while facing away from him, and lifts her legs off the ground, extending them straight out behind her. The man then supports the woman's legs and hips, allowing for deep penetration.

This position can be very stimulating for both partners, as it allows for maximum penetration and skin-to-skin contact. However, it may be difficult to maintain for an extended period of time, and could potentially be uncomfortable for the woman's legs and hips.

2. The "Lusty Leg" position

The Lusty Leg position is a variation of the traditional "Doggy Style" position that allows for deeper penetration and more intense sensations. The woman kneels on all fours while the man enters her from behind, holding onto her hips for support. The woman then lifts one leg off the ground and extends it straight back, allowing the man to penetrate even deeper.

This position can be very pleasurable for both partners, as it allows for maximum penetration and stimulation of the G-spot. However, it may require a higher level of flexibility and balance, and could potentially be uncomfortable for the woman's extended leg.

3. The "Man in the Wheelbarrow" position

The Man in the Wheelbarrow position is a fun and playful position that requires a significant amount of strength and coordination. The woman kneels on all fours while the man stands behind her, holding onto her legs and lifting her off the ground. The woman then walks forward on her hands, while the man supports her weight and thrusts.

This position can be very exhilarating and playful, and allows for deep penetration and a different angle of entry. However, it may require a higher level of strength and coordination, and could potentially be uncomfortable or even dangerous if not executed properly.

4. The "Wheelbarrow" position

The Wheelbarrow position is a variation of the Man in the Wheelbarrow position that requires even more strength and coordination. The woman kneels on all fours while the man stands behind her, holding onto her legs and lifting her off the ground. The woman then straightens her arms and lifts her body into a handstand, while the man supports her weight and thrusts.

This position can be incredibly intense and exciting, and allows for deep penetration and a unique angle of entry. However, it should only be attempted by couples who are both comfortable with the idea, and who have the necessary strength and coordination to execute it safely.

5. The "Cow's Mouth" position

The Cow's Mouth position is a unique and challenging position that requires a high level of flexibility and balance. The woman lies on her back with her legs straight up in the air, while the man kneels between her legs and enters her. The woman then lowers her legs and brings them down to either side of the man's head, creating a "mouth" shape.

This position can be incredibly stimulating for both partners, as it allows for deep penetration and intimate contact. However, it is important to approach this position with caution and communicate with your partner throughout to ensure safety and comfort.

To perform the Cow's Mouth position, start by lying on your back with your legs straight up in the air. Your partner can then kneel between your legs and enter you. As you lower your legs, guide them down to either side of your partner's head, creating a "mouth" shape.

Once in this position, you and your partner can experiment with different movements and angles to find what feels best. You may want to try rocking back and forth or side to side, or your partner may want to lean forward or back to adjust the angle of penetration.

It is important to remember that the Cow's Mouth position requires a high level of flexibility and balance, and it may not be suitable for everyone. If you or your partner feel any discomfort or pain, it is important to stop and try a different position.

6. The "Catherine Wheel" Position

The Catherine Wheel position is an advanced position that requires a great deal of strength and flexibility. This position involves the woman lying on her back with her legs spread wide apart, while the man kneels between her legs and enters her. The woman then lifts her legs up and over her head, allowing the man to penetrate deeply.

This position can be incredibly stimulating for both partners, as it allows for deep penetration and a high level of intimacy. However, it is important to approach this position with caution and communicate with your partner throughout to ensure safety and comfort.

To perform the Catherine Wheel position, start by lying on your back with your legs spread wide apart. Your partner can then kneel between your legs and enter you. As you lift your legs up and over your head, your partner can hold onto your ankles for support.

Once in this position, you and your partner can experiment with different movements and angles to find what feels best. You may want to try rocking back and forth or side to side, or your partner may want to lean forward or back to adjust the angle of penetration.

It is important to remember that the Catherine Wheel position requires a great deal of strength and flexibility, and it may not be suitable for everyone. If you or your partner feel any discomfort or pain, it is important to stop and try a different position.

Conclusion

Exploring different sexual positions and techniques can be an exciting and intimate way to connect with your partner. From the basic positions like the Missionary and Doggy Style, to more advanced positions like the Lusty Leg and Catherine Wheel, there are a wide range of options available to couples.

It is important to approach these positions with caution and communicate with your partner throughout to ensure safety and comfort. Additionally, it is important to remember that not all positions will be suitable for everyone, and it is okay to experiment and find what works best for you and your partner.

Ultimately, the most important aspect of any sexual experience is the connection and intimacy between partners. By exploring different positions and techniques, you and your partner can deepen your connection and enhance your overall sexual experience.

Chapter 6

Emotional and Spiritual Aspects of Intimacy

Intimacy is more than just a physical act, it is a profound emotional and spiritual connection between two people. In this chapter, we will explore the emotional and spiritual aspects of intimacy and how they can deepen your connection with your partner.

Building a Deeper Connection with Your Partner

Intimacy is all about building a deeper connection with your partner. This connection is built on trust, communication, and emotional openness. It is essential to cultivate a safe and supportive environment where both partners can feel comfortable expressing their emotions and desires.

One way to build a deeper connection with your partner is through touch. Touch is a powerful way to communicate love, affection, and intimacy. It can help to create a sense of safety and trust between partners, and can also help to reduce stress and anxiety.

Another way to build a deeper connection with your partner is through communication. Communication is essential for a healthy relationship, both inside and outside of the bedroom. It is essential to be open and honest with your partner about your needs and desires, as well as your fears and insecurities.

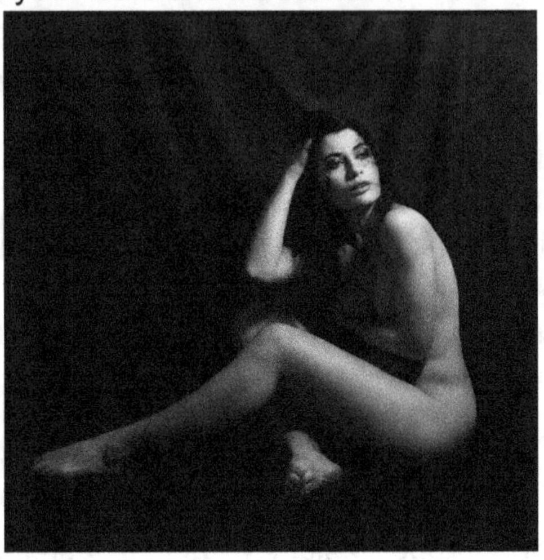

Understanding the Role of Emotions in Lovemaking

Emotions play a crucial role in lovemaking. They can enhance the experience and deepen the connection between partners. However, they can also be a barrier to intimacy if they are not addressed.

One common emotion that can get in the way of intimacy is anxiety. Anxiety can be caused by a variety of factors, including performance anxiety, body image issues, and fear of rejection. It is essential to address these underlying issues and work through them with your partner to build a deeper connection.

Another common emotion that can get in the way of intimacy is shame. Shame can be caused by past experiences, cultural conditioning, or personal beliefs. It is essential to acknowledge and address feelings of shame with your partner, as they can prevent you from fully engaging in intimacy.

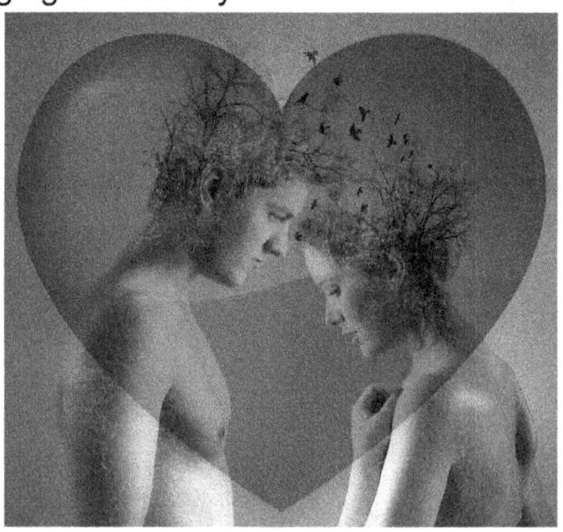

Cultivating Mindfulness and Presence

Mindfulness and presence are essential components of intimacy. Being present in the moment and fully engaged with your partner can enhance the experience and deepen the connection between partners.

One way to cultivate mindfulness and presence is through meditation. Meditation can help to quiet the mind, reduce stress and anxiety, and cultivate a sense of presence and awareness. It can also help to build a deeper connection with your partner by fostering a sense of empathy and compassion.

Incorporating Spiritual Practices into Your Intimate Life

Spiritual practices can be a powerful way to deepen the emotional and spiritual connection between partners. These practices can include anything from prayer and meditation to tantra and yoga.

One popular spiritual practice for couples is tantra. Tantra is an ancient spiritual practice that emphasizes the integration of mind, body, and spirit. It can help to deepen the connection between partners by cultivating a sense of presence, intimacy, and empathy.

Another spiritual practice that can enhance intimacy is yoga. Yoga is a physical and spiritual practice that can help to reduce stress and anxiety, increase flexibility and strength, and cultivate a sense of mindfulness and presence.

Conclusion

Intimacy is more than just a physical act; it is a profound emotional and spiritual connection between two people. By building a deeper connection with your partner, understanding the role of emotions in lovemaking, cultivating mindfulness and presence, and incorporating spiritual practices into your intimate life, you can enhance the experience and deepen your connection with your partner.

Chapter 7

Troubleshooting Common Challenges

Intimate relationships can be incredibly rewarding, but they are not without their challenges. Even with the best intentions and preparation, couples may encounter obstacles during lovemaking that can hinder their ability to connect fully. This chapter will address some common challenges that couples may face and offer practical solutions to overcome them.

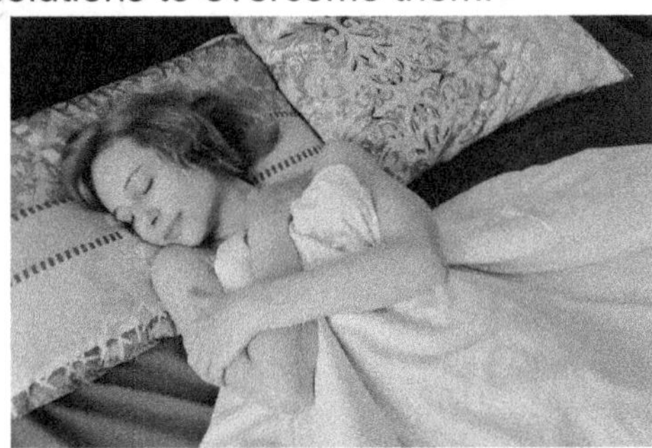

Overcoming difficulties with positioning

One of the most common challenges couples face is finding the right positions that work for them. Each partner may have different preferences or physical limitations that can make certain positions uncomfortable or impractical. In these situations, it is important to communicate openly and honestly with your partner. Be willing to experiment with different positions and take the time to explore each other's bodies to find what works best.

If one partner experiences discomfort or pain during a particular position, it may be necessary to modify or avoid that position altogether. This does not mean that you cannot have a fulfilling and enjoyable sex life. Instead, focus on finding other positions that provide similar stimulation or try incorporating other forms of intimacy, such as kissing, touching, or massage.

Addressing physical discomfort or pain

Physical discomfort or pain during lovemaking is another common challenge that couples may encounter. This can be caused by a variety of factors, such as injury, illness, or tension in the body. It is important to listen to your body and communicate any discomfort or pain to your partner. Ignoring these sensations can lead to further discomfort and potential injury.

If you experience discomfort or pain, take a break from lovemaking and try some gentle stretches or relaxation techniques to release any tension in your body. If the pain persists, consider seeing a healthcare provider to rule out any underlying medical conditions.

Managing emotional challenges or concerns

Intimacy is not just physical; it also involves emotional vulnerability and trust. This can make it challenging for some individuals to fully let go and enjoy the experience. Common emotional challenges that couples may face include anxiety, fear, shame, or past trauma.

It is important to create a safe and supportive environment for your partner to express their feelings and concerns. Be willing to listen without judgment and offer reassurance and encouragement. Consider seeking the support of a therapist or counselor who specializes in sexual health and relationships if these challenges persist.

Maintaining intimacy over time

Maintaining intimacy over time can be challenging as couples navigate the ups and downs of life. Busy schedules, stress, and life changes can all take a toll on intimacy. To maintain a strong connection with your partner, it is important to prioritize intimacy and make time for it regularly.

This can be as simple as setting aside time for a date night, cuddling, or having a conversation about your sexual desires and needs. Don't be afraid to try new things or incorporate different forms of intimacy, such as sensual massage, role-playing, or trying new positions.

In conclusion, overcoming common challenges in intimate relationships requires open communication, a willingness to experiment, and a commitment to maintaining intimacy over time. By addressing these challenges head-on and seeking the support you need, you can build a stronger and more fulfilling connection with your partner.

Chapter 8

Conclusion and Next Steps

In this book, we have explored the ancient art of the Kama Sutra and how it can enhance intimacy between couples. We have covered basic, intermediate, and advanced sexual positions and techniques, as well as emotional and spiritual aspects of intimacy. Additionally, we have provided tips for troubleshooting common challenges that couples may face.

In conclusion, we hope that this book has been a helpful guide for couples looking to deepen their intimacy and explore new dimensions of pleasure. By incorporating the principles and techniques of the Kama Sutra into your intimate life, you and your partner can create a deeper connection and experience heightened physical and emotional pleasure.

If you want to continue your study and exploration of the Kama Sutra, we recommend further reading on the topic. Some recommended resources include:

- "The Complete Kama Sutra: The First Unabridged Modern Translation of the Classic Indian Text" by Alain Daniélou - This is a comprehensive translation of the Kama Sutra that provides detailed descriptions and illustrations of various positions and techniques.

☐ "The Kama Sutra Workbook: A Guide to the Art of Love" by Anne Hooper - This workbook provides step-by-step instructions for practicing the Kama Sutra, as well as exercises and techniques for enhancing intimacy.

"The Book of Erotic Fantasy" by Gwendolyn F.M. Kestrel and Duncan Scott - This book offers a modern interpretation of the Kama Sutra, with illustrations and descriptions of various sexual positions and techniques.

"Tantric Sex: The Fast Track Path to Sexual Bliss" by Diana Richardson - This book explores the principles of tantra and how they can enhance intimacy and pleasure.

As you continue your exploration of the Kama Sutra and other resources for enhancing intimacy, remember to communicate openly and honestly with your partner. Practice mindfulness and presence during intimate moments, and remain patient and compassionate as you navigate any challenges that may arise.

In closing, we encourage you to continue deepening your intimacy with your partner and exploring the many dimensions of pleasure that the Kama Sutra has to offer. By doing so, you can create a more fulfilling and satisfying intimate life for both you and your partner.